Fun Fitness for Families

How to Exercise, Eat Right, and Lose Weight, so You Can Build Self-Esteem and be Great!

Jim Steffen

Published by Jellie Publications
Findlay, OH

Printed in the United States of America

Library of Congress Catalog Card Number:
2005937756

ISBN: 0-9776367-0-4

Text editing by Julie Klein and Dyan Steffen
Cover by Hogrefe Illustration & Design

Table of Contents

Dedicated to my wife, Dyan. This book wouldn't have happened without you.

FOREWORD

Growing up as a kid my parents made sure to instill in me the importance of eating my fruits and vegetables and getting outside to get plenty of fresh air and exercise. I can remember mom saying, "It is a beautiful day outside, turn that TV off and get out there." We played all of the backyard games; football, baseball, and basketball. Riding our bikes, hiking, camping, and fishing also kept us very active.

I carried my athleticism and healthy eating with me to college. That is were I found the freedom and easy access to unhealthy foods which fueled some unhealthy habits. Over that freshman year I gained the famed "freshman fifteen" pounds.

As a sophomore in college, enrolled in the Air Force ROTC program, I exercised and watched what foods I ate. I was trying to "make weight" for the Air Force and found that my workouts and diligence in the cafeteria was paying off. I was six foot one and weighed 204 pounds. I was feeling good about myself and my physical abilities. At the end of that semester, however, I found out that I probably would not be able to loose enough weight to be able to fly F-16's. I decided to leave the ROTC program prior to a long term commitment. This would prove to be a costly mistake.

Upon leaving the program I found that I was not nearly as motivated to continue my strict workouts and I began to eat foods that were not healthy choices. My biggest mistake was that I thought I could enjoy late night fast food with my buddies without any consequences. Seven months later I found that my overindulgence in late night fast food had turned my 204 pound body into a 286 pound body (gaining the weight of my six year old daughter and three year old son combined). That's 82 pounds for those of you doing the math. Let me assure you that the weight gain was not the result of large muscle mass. It was, in fact, large amounts of FAT! I'm not sure what I had expected. For seven months I ventured to Burger King between 11:30 PM and midnight and ate two Whoppers and two large fries. No, that is not a misprint. Yes, it occurred more than four times per week. And on nights where Burger King was not the restaurant of choice, there was pizza, crazy bread, garlic cheese bread, or thirty-five cent burger night at McDonald's (you could get ten burgers for $3.50!).

I graduated after some see-saw battles with weight gain and weight loss. I entered my first job, lost weight to get married, and then gained weight back. The first year of my marriage to Lisa found me learning to eat every meal filled with vegetables and fruits again for the first time since I left home to go to college. Talk about a tough adjustment. I was missing the tastes of all of those fast foods and junk I had grown accustomed to. I began to work with Jim when he taught aerobics at Hard Bodies Gym in Findlay. I would attend his classes for a few months until he left to pursue his career in Chicago and San Diego.

I had had some success with the aerobics and the healthier eating I was doing. However, that trend would not last. I found with my job, I would arrive home earlier than Lisa giving me time for a salty snack without her being any the wiser. I also began my new habit of sitting in my rocking chair and turning on the TV. I was reliving my college days all over again. Needless to say these poor health choices caused my weight to continue to rise. I continued to look and feel terrible. It wasn't until I was wearing 46 inch pants and weighing 297 pounds (three short of 300) that I realized I was slowly pushing myself to an early grave.

God had a hand in what happened next. Jim returned to the Findlay area and he and I began to train together. I slowly began to learn all of the lifting techniques and exercise tips that he had learned from some of the top training facilities in the country.

When Jim opened his first gym (a two car garage behind his house), I moved my morning workouts to his gym. I was one of the first clients he put on the ball as he was developing Jim's Boga. I thought he was crazy. "You want me to stand on that ball and do what?" I was apprehensive at first to try the ball, but I had experienced such success with Jim and his workouts (I had lost 40 pounds and three inches off my stomach) that I was willing to try the ball. After patience, practice, and a few spills onto the floor, I was able to stand on the ball on my own. I could feel my stomach muscles (what Jim calls your core strength) working to keep me on the ball. I was getting stronger just using the weight of my body as resistance.

After working with Jim for a few years, I was able to develop some of my own discipline and have found an exercise program that works for me. As of today, I have been able to increase my cardiovascular and physical strength. Applying proper nutrition has helped to reduce my weight and in turn lowered my percentages for weight related illnesses.

Like Jim states in the start of Chapter 2, I still enjoy unhealthy foods on occasion. They are not however the mainstay of my diet like they once were. I use Saturdays to eat the foods I like, even the really unhealthy ones. I use moderation and make wise choices the other days of the week. There is no quick fix out there. You cannot lose weight without exercising and watching what you put in your mouth. You need to move more. That is what I like about Jim's book. He has designed activities that you can do anywhere, anytime. He teaches you to use juggling toys that you can take with you anywhere.

Kids need guidance in all aspects of their lives. We teach them everything. We need to teach them the benefits of healthy eating and exercise. Lisa makes sure that our family has fruits and vegetables at all of our meals. Our kids are great eaters and try different foods. We still enjoy occasional trips out for fast food or ice cream but we do it in moderation. We also limit the amount of TV our kids can watch each day. In order to turn this obesity trend around, we must model and teach our children healthy eating and exercise habits. We as adults need to be role models for our children and Jim's book "Fun Fitness for Families" has given us a blue print to use to be those role models.

The text is an easy read and the book is packed full of pictures and descriptions. So even if you have never been in a gym before, you can follow the programs and teach kids to follow them too. There are various levels of fitness that Jim talks about in this book. It doesn't matter which level you start at, as long as you start. There is nothing more damaging to your health than inactivity and heavy eating. One push up is better than none. Jim sums it up in Chapter 10 when he says, "Make the change today; don't wait."

Read this book and put the plan in motion. Get "Fit to Achieve" everything you have dreamed about. You can do it and you can help a child in your life learn the benefits of healthy eating and exercise.

Let's "Dig in!"

Kevin Haught
Principal, Arlington Elementary School

INTRODUCTION

The prevalence of childhood obesity is becoming a major problem in the United States. Approximately 15 percent of children ages 6 to 11 are overweight, and studies show that someone who's obese between the ages of 10 and 13 has an 80 percent chance of becoming an obese adult. Overall, 25 to 30 percent of children are affected. Obesity puts these children at risk for myriad health problems including asthma, hypertension and other cardiac risk factors, orthopedic problems, diabetes, and psychological/psychiatric issues such as poor self-esteem and depression. Type 2 diabetes is on the rise in children and The Center for Disease Control is now predicting (assuming current trends continue) that one out of every three babies born today will develop diabetes at some point in his life. This may be the first generation in the US to have a shorter life expectancy than their parents' generation. For the child, obesity can be devastating, not only physically, but also emotionally.

Hormonal and genetic factors are rarely the cause of childhood obesity. It is typically caused by inactivity and improper diet/overeating. Parents need to take control of this situation. I wrote this book to motivate parents to start an exercise program and healthy eating lifestyle. How can you tell your child to stop eating junk food and to get off the couch if you're not doing those things too? A recent *Parents* magazine poll indicated that 51% of parents haven't worked out in years. Parents play a crucial role in helping children develop healthy habits, control weight, and feel good.

The Fun Fitness Program I've developed is an enthusiastic solution for families who need some basic instruction to get started on the right path to exercise and healthy eating. You and your children will have hours of family fun as you learn a whole new exciting concept of exercise.

I've also developed a "5 STEPP" success program that you can apply to your new healthy lifestyle. This program will help you set both short-term and long-term attainable goals. These steps will help you stay motivated as you begin your new lifestyle. You and your children will be able to learn and apply these same concepts to other goals in life as well.

Now let's get started and soon you and your family will be "Fit to Achieve" all of your biggest dreams!

CHAPTER 1

Dig In – With Optimism

"Perpetual optimism is a force multiplier."
- Colin Powell

When I played high school basketball in Findlay, OH in 1987 I had a coach named Al Baker. Coach Baker was our defensive coach. We knew when coach blew the whistle and told us to line up and face him, we were about to be in for some pain. Coach Baker would first demonstrate how he wanted the defensive shuffle done: telling us to "get low with your rear down, wide stance, arms up and out." Coach would then blow the whistle and point to the left, right, forward, backward, and so on. After a few minutes of the dreaded defensive shuffle and with our leg muscles burning, we would start to stand up, our arms would come down, and our stances closed together. Coach would blow the whistle again and, shaking his head, tell us our stance was getting sloppy and lackadaisical, and that we needed to be low for balance, to get down and DIG IN.

Years later reflecting on Coach Baker's defensive shuffle drill, I decided that I didn't want to go through life sloppy, lackadaisical, and off balance; I wanted to live life sharp, motivated, and balanced. I wanted to **dig in**! **I made exercise and nutrition a daily part of my life. And you can too. My goal is to motivate you to embark on a *lifestyle* of exercise and healthy, moderate eating.**

Everyone is familiar with the benefits of regular exercise and good nutrition: stronger bones and more lean muscle, lower cholesterol and blood pressure, decreased body fat, pain relief to arthritic joints, regulation of blood sugar for diabetes and many more. The benefits that really get me excited are the increased energy level and altered attitude a healthy lifestyle affords us. Exercise and healthy eating makes you feel better all around; it gives you a sense of well-being, and as a result you feel happiness and joy. You feel better about yourself and surprisingly start to feel better about a lot of other things in life too. Before you know it, you'll be "Fit to Achieve" anything.

I own Jim's Gym Family Fitness in Findlay, Ohio. When members join my gym, the first thing I like to stress is optimism, what I call the "Big O." According to Webster's, if you're optimistic, you have the tendency to take the most hopeful view of matters and believe good things will happen. This attitude is critical to success in a fitness program and in overcoming any of life's obstacles. In fact, Sir Winston Churchill said, "For myself, I'm an optimist. It does not seem to be of much use being anything else." Lucille Ball once said, "One of the things I learned the hard way was that it doesn't pay to get discouraged. Keeping busy and making optimism a way of life can restore your faith in yourself." Successful people throughout history, as well as people today in my gym, have a lot of the "Big O" in common.

I've always had an optimistic view. For example, when I was 12 years old I received a synthetic leather indoor/outdoor basketball for Christmas. I lived for basketball, but growing up in Ohio it was hard to play in the snow covered driveway until sometime in March. So I did everything I could indoors – I learned how to spin it on my finger and practiced dribbling in the basement. I loved my pristine, new basketball and even slept with the ball sometimes! I repeatedly told my family how much I loved my basketball and how it was going to be an indoor ball only, so it would stay new and not lose its dimpled texture.

Then, the weather changed. Late in March on a warm Saturday afternoon, my brother John and I played basketball outside in the driveway for hours with my brand new synthetic leather basketball. It took a beating that afternoon, getting wet in mud puddles and scraping against the rough asphalt. As the Ohio State Buckeyes (me) were winning in double overtime against the Indiana Hoosiers (John), my mom called us in for dinner. Suddenly, I realized that I couldn't even take my formerly perfect basketball into the house because it was now dirty, wet, and scraped. No dimples covering this ball anymore. My heart sank some as I realized it would never be the same again. As I sat down to dinner with my family, I told everyone I liked my ball better now that it was broken in. Deep in my heart, I missed the look and feel of the new ball, but I liked to look at things optimistically – even then. A brand new ball doesn't help a 12 year-old kid's basketball skills improve. A battered, scuffed ball shows dedicated practice and improved skills. Ultimately, something good came out of the situation. I spent countless happy hours in the driveway practicing with that ball and eventually played basketball for Findlay High School and, later, the University of Findlay. To this day, my family jokes about my new basketball and my optimistic attitude.

Owning my own fitness center, I encounter numerous people who start an exercise program, but for various reasons don't stick to it. Those members who join with an optimistic attitude and a high degree of certainty that they will prevail have a much higher success rate than those that hold a pessimistic attitude. I have many experiences of optimistic members that might not be the most athletically skilled, but who have had great results nonetheless. I believe their optimism made the difference.

One gloomy January day, I was talking at the smoothie bar with one of my members, Cindy. Cindy had seen great results – decreased body fat and increased energy – but she was having one of "those" days. She shared that she feared she was losing motivation and wondered what she could do to get back on track. As we started talking, another member, Father Joe Weigman, struggled to get on the treadmill. Father Joe has multiple sclerosis. He uses a wheelchair, but can walk with the assistance of a walker. When Joe gets on a treadmill, he has to hang on, lean into it, and it takes every bit of his strength and energy to walk at 0.5 mph. Since Joe had joined the gym 3 months earlier, his treadmill record was 5 minutes.

For those of you who are unfamiliar with treadmills, the average person usually walks between 3 – 4.5 mph for 30 – 60 minutes. As Cindy and I were talking, Joe came up behind us in his wheelchair and with an earsplitting grin said, "Six minutes today, Jim!"

The optimism of that one statement was contagious. As Joe wheeled away, Cindy paused in deep thought. She looked at me and said, "Now that's an optimistic attitude. I will never grumble about not being motivated to exercise again." Author and educator Nicholas Murray Butler said, "Optimism is the foundation of courage." Father Joe radiates courage every time he comes through the doors for another work-out.

If you've wanted to start an exercise program, have been putting it off for some reason, or have made excuses for not exercising, then remember Father Joe. Have optimism! When you start your exercise program or any new venture in life and things aren't happening as fast as you would like, remember the Big O – be optimistic and dig in!

CHAPTER 2

SACRIFICE: Achievement is born of great sacrifice

"Sweat plus sacrifice equals success."

- Charles Finley

While Optimism is an essential factor to success, I've also identified 5 other key components for creating success in life. Let's start with the first step in my 5 STEPP Success Program: Sacrifice. Sacrifice is the giving up of one thing for the sake of another. This is a very important step when you decide to begin an exercise program. You can also apply this to any endeavor you want to achieve in your life. Sometimes you have to let go of favorite things in order to achieve a goal. Author Napoleon Hill said, "Great achievement is usually born of great sacrifice, and is never the result of selfishness."

I've been in the exercise industry since 1991 and the biggest excuse I hear for not being able to exercise is time constraints. If you want something badly enough, like an old friend of mine used to say, "make it happen!" Dr. C.C. Albert wrote this about the use of time, "It might be wise for us to take a little inventory of our resources as to time and review our habits of using it." So, let's review our time:
168 hours in each week.
56 of them we spend in sleep.
40 of them we spend at work.
17.5 of them we spend eating meals.
2 of them in church/prayer time.

We have left 52.5 hours a week for family, recreation, chores/errands, and yes, even exercise. There's definitely time in the week to exercise if it is made a priority. It becomes even easier to get in your exercise time if you combine exercise and family time by using the Fun Fitness Program for the entire family.

During my college years, I started to get really serious about my exercise and eating program. All my college friends were staying out late, going to parties and getting in at 1:00 a.m., eating cheeseburgers and fries and then going right to bed. I knew if I wanted to live that lifestyle, my 8:00 a.m. workouts would suffer. The food they were putting in their bodies was enough to make even the elite professional athlete put on extra, unhealthy body fat. Don't get me wrong! I had a fun college experience and didn't eat great all the time, but I made sacrifices and moderate decisions that enabled me to exercise. By doing so, I could maintain a healthy physical body. The energy and confidence I reaped helped me with all aspects of life.

So what kind of sacrifice am I talking about? Tape your favorite show at night, so you can get to bed 1 hour earlier. You can then rise refreshed and ready to get in your 30 - 60 minutes of exercise. Sacrifice that unneeded dessert after dinner or that late night snack that does absolutely zero for your physical and mental well-being. Serve fresh fruit for dessert instead of something high in fat or you can still pick a day (or two if you use moderation) and splurge with your favorite foods. By exercising and eating right daily, those splurge days should have little effect on your ultimate goal of a healthy lifestyle. You may need to sacrifice some of the quick, pre-packaged foods and take the time to prepare healthier alternatives. Don't buy the sugary snacks for your children. Take the extra time to peel an apple or prepare a healthy snack for the after school munchies. Ban the open bag of potato chips on the couch.

I'm a firm believer in 7 to 8 hours of sleep a night. Getting proper sleep and getting up a little earlier than usual gives you time to complete your exercise program and eat breakfast to rev up that metabolism for the day. Don't get me wrong, anytime of the day is great to exercise; I just happen to be a morning person. Just find a time that works best for you and enjoy your journey of exercise.

Remember the words from Vince Lombardi, "...if you are willing to sacrifice the little things in life and pay the price for the things that are worthwhile, it can be done."

CHAPTER 3

TARGET: Set your goals and aim high

"The big secret in life is that there is no big secret. Whatever your goal, you can get there if you're willing to work."
- Oprah Winfrey

The second step in my 5 STEPP Success Program for achieving unlimited results is to establish a Target. You need to have an objective to work towards, so set a goal and aim high. When a new member joins my fitness center, the first thing I do is set a goal with that person.

I take their circumference measurements. Using calipers, I take body composition (body fat) and then I weigh them. Unless you're involved in a competitive sport, the majority of people's goals are similar when starting an exercise program. They, of course, want to lose weight. They want to tone up problem areas: arms, thighs and stomach. And if possible, they want to have more energy, because they tend to be tired a lot. Or their doctor recommended them to exercise for a specific health problem - joint pain, high cholesterol, blood pressure, etc.

Together we set short-term and long-term goals. An average healthy range for males is between 12% - 18% body fat and for females it's between 16% - 25% body fat. **For example, a realistic short-term goal for a 5'5" woman who weighs 160 pounds and has 32% body fat would be 1- 3 percent of body fat loss every 8 weeks.**

Notice that I like to set body fat loss goals rather than weight loss goals, especially the first 3 to 4 months of a new exercise program. If you weigh-in all the time, it could get discouraging. The positive stress you're taking your body through will result in some calorie burning muscle gain. Muscle is denser than fat and it may appear that you aren't losing at all or are even gaining weight. I've seen far too many people drop out of a program because they got addicted to the scale and didn't lose the weight they wanted. (Be patient, we'll talk about this more later.)

If you can meet your short-term goals in 8 week increments, this gives you hope to reach the long-term goal that you set for yourself. Your long-term goal could take anywhere from 12 - 24 months to achieve. Of course, the timeframe depends on what your goals are and how much body fat/weight you have to lose. If it took you years to gain this excess fat, you'll need time to lose it. Author Saul Bellow said, "Whoever wants to reach a distant goal must take small steps." So start with those small steps and enjoy your new journey of exercise and healthy eating; it's fun!

While you are working towards your target, remember the immediate benefits you get from exercise: the energy you'll have, the increased blood flow which carries vital oxygen and nutrients to all parts of your body, the confidence and sense of well-being you'll feel from the accomplishment of sticking with and excelling at your program, the impact you are making in your children's lives, and the fun you are now having together.

The rate of success with my members is much higher if they set short-term and long-term goals right away. I like to look at it like you're starting a new business. Make a 1 - 2 year business plan by writing down all accomplishments and goals you want to achieve in that time period. It is important to actually write down your goals rather than just have goals in mind. Make sure you write down the exact dates you want to achieve them. Make copies of your goals and keep them in your wallet or purse, so you can read them constantly. Stick them to your mirror, so you see them in the morning. Put them on your office desk and read it daily. I personally like to put them on the visor of my car, so I can read them before I start the car. Before you know it, your exercise lifestyle "business" will flourish. It's up to you if you want to succeed, so aim high, but realistically.

Following is a measurement and goal sheet you can fill out as well as some examples of realistic goal-setting. Get started by finding someone to take your body fat. Local health clubs may do it for free the first time. Then you can go back every 8 weeks and get re-evaluated. They probably will charge you after the first time, but it is well worth it. I like caliper testing the best. If you have a scale that tests body fat, that will do. I recommend these goals only be re-evaluated every 8 weeks. If you want to test them every 6 weeks, that is fine. Just don't get discouraged if things aren't happening as fast as you want. Your number one priority is making a lifestyle commitment to exercise and healthy moderate eating! And I know you can do it! I would also recommend having all of the family members evaluated, so you're all doing this together as a family.

Name _____

Starting Date_____

Body Fat Percentage_____

Weight_____

Circumference Measurements:

Arm extended palm up   Right_____   Left_____

Waist (women, thinnest part, men, around belly button) _____

Hips (feet together, around widest point) _____

Thighs   Right_____   Left_____

After you have your measurements, you can write out your fitness goals. Remember, these goals can always be modified as you progress through the year. Again, you want to keep the goals realistic, but yet challenging. A sample of a 1 ½ year fitness plan follows. I suggest buying a journal or binder note pad in which to record your goals and work-out notes or you can copy the blank fitness plan included.

Sample Fitness Plan

Elaine Smith
Starting Date: Jan 1st
Body Fat: 33%
Weight: 170

Goal: Lose 40 lbs and get down to 20% body fat

1) By March 1st, I will have 31% body fat. I will exercise at least 3 times a week for 30 to 60 minutes.   I will take walks with my children in the evenings at least twice a week. I will only drink 1 Coke a day instead of 3.   I'll reduce the amount of juice and soda pop my children consume. I'll start eating breakfast every morning and I'll ensure my children are eating breakfast too.

2) By May 1st, I will be 29%. Weight goal, 160 lbs. No more fast food and I'm only serving/having dessert two times a week (cut back from 4). I'm walking with my children and going to the park at least three times per week.

3) By July 1st, 26%. Weight goal 150 lbs. I will start working out 5 days a week and include my children in these work-outs. Eliminate soda pop completely for me and children.

4) By September 1st, 24% Weight goal 145

5) By November 1st, 22% Weight goal 140

6) By January 1st of next year, 21% Weight 135

7) By March 1st, 20% Weight 130

8) By May 1st, 19% Weight is perfect

9) By July 1st, 18% Weight is perfect

Fitness Plan Template

Name _____

Starting Date_____

Body Fat Percentage_____

Weight_____

Overall Goal

_____

Goal to be reached in 8 weeks

_____

on _____ (date)

Exercise targets:

Eating changes:

Goal to be reached in 8 weeks

_____

on _____ (date)

Exercise targets:

Eating changes:

Goal to be reached in 8 weeks

_____

on _____ (date)

Exercise targets:

Eating changes:

Goal to be reached in 8 weeks

_____

on _____ (date)

Exercise targets:

Eating changes:

Goal to be reached in 8 weeks

_____

on _____ (date)

Exercise targets:

Eating changes:

Again, these are samples, but hopefully it gives you some ideas to get started. Just writing these goals down on paper and reading them over daily will help your success rate immensely. Notice during the first 4 months that Elaine didn't set a weight goal. Remember what I said about your body responding with some lean muscle gain when you start to exercise, especially the first few months. This is exciting and you'll start to notice your body toning up. Since muscle is more dense than fat, you shouldn't expect to see the pounds come off immediately. Please don't get addicted to weighing in, but you can get addicted to your hour of exercise a day!

I bet you're saying, "Ok, Jim I have my goals written down, now what do I do?" Well, I'm glad you asked. Keep reading and you'll learn all the basic instructions you need from yours truly, America's Fun Fitness Coach.

CHAPTER 4

ENTHUSIASM: It's contagious

"Nothing great was ever achieved without enthusiasm."

- Ralph Waldo Emerson

I've been personal training and working in health clubs for almost 15 years and one thing I've observed is the more enthusiasm you have about your workout, the more likely you are to succeed. Not only are you more likely to thrive, but also more likely to stick with a lifestyle of exercise. Enthusiasm means lively, intense, or eager interest.   Become passionate about your exercise program and exercise with great fervor. It will make a difference!

For example, I have two friends who joined the gym together -"Beth" and "Jane." Right from the very start, the enthusiasm was evident in Beth. She had a great, positive attitude. Jane was also a very pleasant woman, but she seemed to be somewhat of a pessimist and wasn't really excited about being there. Beth's body fat was around 27% and Jane's body fat was 28%. Both ladies joined my gym for one year. One year later, Beth is at 17% body fat. She comes in every morning with enthusiasm at 5:00 a.m. Because of this enthusiasm and dedication, she has thrived and stayed dedicated to her new healthy lifestyle. Jane, on the other hand, only lasted about eight weeks. She was always grumbling and coming up with excuses for not exercising. Beth and Jane are still good friends and Jane still grumbles to Beth about how tired she feels and how she needs to lose body fat.   Show some enthusiasm and passion, a little fervor and zeal, and you will be surprised at the difference it makes in your commitment, longevity and work ethic at your exercise program, or anything you want to tackle in life.

An enthusiastic attitude will benefit you in all aspects of your life.   I've had countless people work for me over the past 8 years. A lot of them have had exercise physiology degrees or exercise science certifications from very reputable colleges and organizations, but they lacked enthusiasm.   A couple of years ago, I decided to hire my younger sister Jenny. Jenny had just graduated with an undergraduate degree in Art.   She is in good shape, exercises and stays active, so I taught her the basic techniques of resistance training, flexibility, monitoring members' heart rates during cardio-respiratory training, etc.

And I soon came to realize that Jenny has something more valuable than any advanced degree in the fitness field. She has enthusiasm. She is a real person with deep, genuine enthusiasm. Members change their schedules to exercise when she is working. She is now in charge of the seniors program at my gym. Because of Jenny's enthusiastic attitude, calling everyone by name, and having a vivacious smile, the seniors program is now one of the busiest and most successful programs at the gym. Jenny creates an atmosphere of enthusiasm and excitement.

According to Dale Carnegie, "Genuine, heartfelt enthusiasm is one of the most potent factors of success in almost any undertaking."   When Mark

Twain was asked the reason for his success, he replied "I was born excited." If anyone was born excited, it was Jenny. And you know the best thing about enthusiasm? Enthusiasm is contagious. It makes the attitude of those around you change, which helps maintain and keep my members coming back into a positive, motivating, and uplifting environment. Jenny's enthusiasm keeps spreading and it can work for you too. Getting your family members excited about fitness and sharing the enthusiasm will get all of you motivated and moving!

William Lyon Phelps, one of the most popular teachers in the history of Yale, said that "one of the chief reasons for success in life is the ability to maintain a daily interest in one's work, to have a chronic enthusiasm; to regard each day as important." So when you commit to a lifestyle of exercise and healthy eating, do it with enthusiasm. Get excited about your new lifestyle; your success rate will be so much higher and you'll enjoy it more along the way.

CHAPTER 5

Patience & Perseverance: No Six Week Abs

> *"Patience and perseverance have a magical*
> *effect before which difficulties disappear*
> *and obstacles vanish."*
> *- John Quincy Adams*

The last two steps in my "5-Stepp Success Fitness Program" are Patience and Perseverance. Patience is calmly tolerating delay and perseverance is to continue on a course of action in spite of difficulty or opposition. I like to group these two together because they have similar characteristics.   Let's face it, we are living in a world where everyone wants quick and easy results that don't take a lot of effort or time. Just look at all the infomercials out there promising "6 Week Abs!," "30 pound loss in six weeks!," "It's as easy as taking a weight loss pill!," etc.

This is not to say the product they're marketing isn't a quality tool, but look closely at the bottom of the screen. You have to get real close to the TV and squint.   For a short time, it usually reads "results may vary." That disclaimer means that if you don't get the results they show on the infomercial when you use this product or machine, it's probably your fault due to either your diet or your lack of additional exercise. There may be value in some of these products, but what I've learned in my fitness experience is, there are NO quick fixes. It takes Patience and Perseverance.

I get numerous people coming into my gym on what I call 6 to 12 week missions. This means they are going on vacation in a couple of months and will be wearing a swimsuit, or their class reunion is right around the corner. And oh, by the way, they usually haven't been physically active in years. They want to drop a quick 30 pounds in two months and they will do anything it takes. I get this scenario frequently, and this is what I tell them:

Depending on how much excess body fat they have to lose (which is usually in excess of 10%), it will likely take much longer than that. If it took you 10 years to put the weight on, it won't come back off in 2 months. Like I said in the goal-setting chapter, if you can lose 1-3% body fat every eight weeks (say they lose 1.5%), you can lose 12% in 16 months with Patience and Perseverance. So from 35% to 23% body fat, you're now in a range where you should be feeling good about your body.

Will you see results in 8 weeks? Of course! You'll feel excellent, you'll have more energy and confidence, and other people will notice your change in attitude; your positive sense of well-being will be evident. You will also see a degree of body fat loss. And with Patience and Perseverance, because you chose this new lifestyle of exercise and healthy, moderate eating, you'll be where you want to be in 12 - 24 months. Remember, the amount of body fat you have will determine the amount of time it takes.

Make a commitment to the long haul and Persevere. Don't settle for the trap of yo-yo dieting in order to meet short-term goals. Know that the quick-fix fad diet will not provide the long term healthy lifestyle you deserve. Former Prime Minister of England Benjamin Disraeli said, "Through perseverance many people win success out of what seemed destined to be certain failure."

I have another member who I'll call Ed. Ed is fifty years old and has been at my gym for about 1 month. He works out 3 - 4 times a week and hasn't changed what he eats, but did cut back on portion size. And for the past 3 weeks, he's been complaining about how he isn't losing any weight. So I've had to remind Ed about some basic exercise physiology facts and provide a pep talk:

Ed, remember, you haven't been on a regular exercise program your entire adult life. Give your body a chance to adapt to this new good stress (exercise) from the resistance and cardiovascular training. Your muscles may increase in size a little bit, so the first 3months you may gain 3 - 4 pounds of lean muscle and, remember, 1 pound of muscle is so much more dense than fat. So in the first couple of months if the scale doesn't show any weight loss, I can take your body fat measurement and show that you gained 3 pounds of calorie-burning lean muscle, while losing 4 pounds of fat. 3 pounds of muscle can fit in the palms of both hands put together. In order to hold 4 pounds of fat, you would have to hold it by cradling it like a baby. So, Ed, even though the scale only said 1 pound lost in 2 months, you're doing great. Trust the trainer, and be Patient and Persevere!

Be Patient and Persevere over the 12 month goal we set together. Members tell me repeatedly that they feel much better and have more energy, and their attitudes have changed to be more optimistic. So enjoy your lifestyle change of exercise and continue eating healthy and moderately. Author

Napoleon Hill said, "Patience, persistence, and perspiration make an unbeatable combination for success." And I always follow Benjamin Franklin's advice, "He that can have patience can have what he will."

CHAPTER 6

Move and Eat Less: It's That Simple

> **"I've been on a diet for two weeks and all**
> **I've lost is two weeks**
> **- Totie Fields**

Now that you're excited and motivated to make exercise a part of your lifestyle, let's briefly touch on your eating program, and let's keep it as basic as possible.

I enjoy eating. Let me say that again, I really enjoy eating. I think it goes back to my Greek heritage on my mother's side; food was always a big deal around our house. Mom would cook a variety of her favorite recipes and she would always let us know what time dinner was, so we could eat together as a family. Because Mom knew we would be outside, doing some activity with the neighborhood kids, she was always certain to tell us a time to come in for dinner. It seemed like our house was the house where everyone congregated for kickball, basketball, jumping on the trampoline, playing freeze tag, etc.

Oh yes, I remember those wonderful home cooked meals, the pork and seashells, the stuffed peppers and cabbage, the chili and grilled cheese that made the house smell so good all day, and one of my personal favorites, the city chicken legs (pork on a stick), and how could I forget the traditional fish fry on Fridays that my grandfather, "Papa," caught at the lake. I always got excited about the traditional pizza night, on Sunday (which I still do in my house today). I can remember Mom would only get one large pizza and I would grumble that it wasn't enough. Well, as I look back on it now, I realize it was more than enough. And Mom was always good at putting some kind of vegetable with our meals. I can't leave out the wonderful banana splits smothered with all the different strawberry, chocolate, or caramel toppings, and then topping it off with whipped cream and nuts. I have very fond memories of eating as a child.

The reason I'm describing some of the food I ate as a child is because I want you to see that we ate a variety of different foods, not always the most low-fat. We ate foods that hit all four food groups and our portion sizes weren't out of control. None of us were over-weight. I think this was due primarily to two reasons.

The first reason is that we were always involved in some neighborhood activity, like I said earlier. We were always eager to get outside and do something rather than sit in front of the TV, computer (we didn't even have one in the mid-eighties), or play video games (we only had Atari back then). We spent our summer weekends in Michigan at Clark Lake, so my parents and grandparents always seemed to give us fun activities to do whether it was water skiing, tubing, swimming, catching frogs or turtles, trying to beat my dad in basketball or going for walks at night with flashlights (I could have walked forever with my family at night, what an adventure at age eight).   The important point I'm trying to make here is that my parents were involved in my physical activities (which I viewed as fun games).

The second reason why we didn't put on the extra pounds (that haunts so many kids today) is that we ate a lot of home cooked meals where we had to sit down and take our time and enjoy our eating experience with each other. We weren't eating breakfast on the go or driving thru McDonald's and eating unhealthy food on the run. Sure, there were fast food and ice cream stops, but they weren't an everyday occurrence. Like I said at the beginning, I want to keep this chapter as simple as possible: move more and eat a variety of freshly prepared, smaller-portion meals together as a family.

Remember what I said in the Target chapter, this is a lifestyle change of exercise and healthy moderate eating, so don't expect changes overnight. If you and your children are trying to shed those extra pounds, give yourself 12 to 24 months. Here is my top ten list of small changes you can make in your eating program that will help you lose and keep off that unwanted fat. Try adding one or two of these ideas each week.

1. Try not to snack after dinner. Your body doesn't need that extra energy to get through the evening; you have plenty of nutrients from dinner. If this is asking a lot, just start by cutting your snack in half. That can result in extra pounds dropped over a period of a couple months. If you and your children like to have a snack between meals, that's a perfect time for fruit, a handful of nuts, yogurt - something healthy and nutritious.

2. Balance out each meal. When you look down at your plate, make sure you have a balance of protein, carbohydrates, and some fat. Here is what has been successful with my clients over

the years: 1/3 of your plate should be protein, (eg. chicken, fish, lean red meat, eggs, cottage cheese, tofu). Another 1/3 should be a vegetable (such as spinach, broccoli, asparagus, carrots, etc. Pick your favorites, but make sure you have a variety). The last 1/3 should be a starch (potato, rice, pasta, etc.) I know what some of you are saying right now, Pasta?! Rice?! Potato?! You're not supposed to eat carbs! Wrong. Just don't overeat them and balance them out with the other foods. Remember, moderate, healthy eating. We always eat whole wheat pasta. Trust me, your kids won't notice a difference.

3. Drink more water. I don't count how many glasses I have a day, but I do make a conscious effort to drink water throughout the day. I tell my clients that every time you drink a beverage other than water, you can't have another drink until you've had that much water. For example, if you have 12 ounces of coffee, you can't have another cup until you drink 12 ounces of water. You might be surprised how good you feel and how refreshing water is.

4. Eat breakfast. This doesn't mean a bowl of sugary cereal, although a whole grain cereal is great. Get that metabolism started for the day, get that fire burning. Wake up a little earlier, so you can prepare a breakfast for your family. What a great way to start the day and to get some time in with the family. Remember, sit down and enjoy your meals; eating breakfast on the run is unacceptable.

5. Limit fast food. Try not to get in the habit of eating fast food. Do it maybe once a week, if that. I personally don't eat fast food at all. Go to the supermarket with your children and pick something fresh and healthy you can go home and prepare together. Wow, sounds like fun! I know this takes time, but do it for you and your family's health and well-being.

6. Put your fork down between each bite. We've all heard this before, but it really does make a difference. You eat slower, you won't eat as much, and if you enjoy eating like I do you can savor each bite.

7. No more sugary fruit juice or soda pop. I suggest you eat the fruit instead of drink it; you'll get more vitamins and minerals and add essential fiber to your diet as well. Maybe treat yourself to a soda on pizza night, but limit your intake. Read every label and stay away from products that say "high fructose corn syrup." Be wary of products with a list of ingredients a mile long, most of which are unpronounceable.

8. Don't go to the grocery store hungry. I've done this one too many times and always come back with unneeded junk food.

9. Don't sit down to a meal hungry. If you eat lunch at noon and don't get around to eating dinner until seven, try a healthy mid-afternoon snack, so you aren't famished when you sit down to dinner and end up overeating.

10. Take time to prepare your food. Tape or skip your favorite Sunday and Wednesday night programs so you and your children can plan and prepare healthy meals and snacks. It takes some sacrifice, but it will keep you from making those fast food stops or grabbing those cookies or chips.

I don't know about you, but I am very excited about this lifestyle change of healthy, moderate eating. Don't get discouraged if the pounds don't come off as fast as you would like and you seem to be cheating on your eating goals every other day. Review my FIVE STEPP success program. Circle the "STEPPS" with the big O, OPTIMISM. Then start with SACRIFICE, shoot for a TARGET, aim high, set goals, be as ENTHUSIASTIC and excited about your new program as possible, and have PATIENCE. This is a new life long journey not a short term program. PERSEVERE.   If you run into obstacles along the way, stay focused on your target. Remember what Entrepreneur Joseph Cossman said, "Obstacles are things a person sees when he takes his eyes off his goals."

I'm rooting for you. I know you can do it. The benefits will truly outweigh the extra time and effort you put into it.   I love the quote from painter Thomas Eakins: "Enthusiasm for one's goal lessens the disagreeableness of working toward it." Wow! That gets me excited. I think I'll go have a healthy snack!

CHAPTER 7

THE FUN FITNESS EXERCISE PROGRAMS: Let's
Have Fun

> **"…happiness gives us the energy which
> is the basis of health."**
> **- Henri-Frederic Amiel**

Like the eating chapter, let's also keep this
exercise thing as basic as possible. I've always been
physically active; ever since I can remember I loved
gymnastics and basketball. I can remember
countless hours of shooting baskets or practicing
walking on my hands. So after I graduated from high
school and had three great years on the basketball
team, I continued playing basketball at the YMCA and
also started to lift weights. I then played basketball at
college. I loved the natural high I got from physical
exertion; it made me feel great and it kept my
confidence high.

I like to stress the way exercise makes you feel
more than how it makes you look. However, there
isn't anyone out there among us who wouldn't
psychologically feel better standing in front of a full-
length mirror and noticing more muscle tone and not
as much excess body fat around their midsection.
Remember what I said in the first chapter, the benefits
of exercise I like best are the sense of well being, the
confidence, the optimistic attitude, and the energy.
The by-product of a regular exercise program is the
pounds of fat you will lose.

In my gym, I have the treadmills, elliptical
trainers, recumbent bikes, and all the fancy weight

training machines. This equipment is great; it keeps things exciting and you have a lot of variety. However, you don't need to join a gym (unless of course you live in the Findlay, OH area and can join Jim's Gym!) to be successful making a lifestyle change of exercise. That's what I'm going to show you in this chapter.

Before we begin, go back and memorize my 5 "STEPP" success program. That's what will give you the motivation you need. I've owned Jim's Gym now for 8 years and have been in the industry for 15 years, and it's still amazing to me the number of people who start a program and drop out soon after they start. Statistics show that 50% of people will drop off within the first six months and after that 30 % will follow. This means only 20% of the people who start an exercise program will continue and make it a life long journey. I know it's difficult and takes time and effort, but that's why I'm going to help you.   I'm going to show you a Fun Fitness Program that you can do at home with the whole family. Making exercise fun for you and your children will make it much easier to sustain.

I've personally trained numerous people over the years from ages 4 to 84 and some of them took the instruction and knowledge I gave them and continued a lifestyle of exercise. Unfortunately with a drop-out rate hovering near 80%, many didn't take the advice. One major reason (excuse) for not staying motivated is boredom with exercise. Well, the Fun Fitness Coach is at your beck and call to banish boredom. I'm going to teach you a unique, fun exercise program that is very effective; you just have to do it! Now that you have the 5 "STEPP" success program memorized and you can't wait to wake up tomorrow morning to begin your Fun Fitness Program, let me teach you how to get started.

First of all, consult your doctor before starting this or any exercise program. A clean bill of health is always good for your mental attitude as well. If you have limitations that prevent you from doing any of these exercises or you experience shooting pains that don't feel like muscle fatigue, please stop the program and consult your physician. You will have to make a few minor purchases. You'll need a Swiss exercise ball and a set of juggling balls. Any size of juggling balls will do to get started. You can order regulation size juggling balls off my website funfitnesscoach.com.

What kind of exercise ball should you get? The only ball I use is a Dura-ball Pro. If you ever use one, you'll never want to use anything else. You can also order these from my web page. They are well worth the money and they will last. If you already have a ball, that will do fine. Keep in mind that for some of the more advanced moves, you'll need a firm ball that withstands dynamic resistance.

What size ball is right for you? When you sit on your ball your thighs should be parallel to the floor or a little above parallel. You can get a 45cm, 55cm, 65cm, or 75cm ball. The 55cm and 65cm balls are the most popular. Ball size is determined more by your leg length than your total height. A 55cm can usually be used by the whole family to have hours of fun.

You'll also need to bring an optimistic attitude. With that said, let's DIG IN!

CHAPTER 8

JIM'S BOGA FITNESS PROGRAM

What is Jim's Boga? It is similar to yoga, but it's performed on a ball and is so much more fun! Let me give you a brief history about the Swiss exercise ball. The exercise ball has been around longer than people think. They used the ball in the 1960's for children who had accidents that limited their ability to move or were in body casts for long periods of time, so their muscles wouldn't atrophy. Physical therapists realized that children enjoyed rolling around on the ball and that the ball helped them to regain their muscle tone. The ball has many more benefits. One of the main benefits is that it strengthens your core. Your core muscles are the deep muscles underneath your abdominals that keeps your spine in alignment. Your core is where your power is. When you move your extremities, your core muscles are the first muscles to contract. The stronger your core is, the more strength you'll have to walk, run, jump, hit, throw, swing, or any activity you do in life.

The ball is also great for balance, because it works your stabilizer muscles. Stabilizer muscles are muscles that surround your joints - wrists, elbows, shoulders, spine, hips, knees, ankles, etc. Strengthening stabilizer muscles will help keep you from getting injured. The ball is also one of the most effective tools for creating perfect posture. We all know that America is plagued with back problems. Jim's Boga could possibly be a remedy for back problems or at least it will relieve some of the discomfort.

We're going to start with The Awakening, which is the warm-up in Jim's Boga Fitness Program. It can last as long as you like, I usually do it for 10 minutes, but you can do it as long as you want. It stretches out the whole body and makes you feel great, and it's loads of fun for the whole family! Just doing 10 to 15 minutes of The Awakening every day can be great for your back and flexibility.

Before we begin learning the positions, please review the list below:

1. Make sure you have a lot of space. Move all tables and chairs out of the way and make sure the surface is not slippery; carpet is great.

2. You should be inhaling deeply through your nose and exhaling through your mouth or back out your nose. Just make sure throughout Jim's Boga, you keep a constant breath, expanding those lungs, delivering a rich supply of oxygen to your working muscles. Remember your blood stream carries the nutrients and oxygen to your working muscles. This blood will get deep in the joints and will keep them healthy.

3. If you get dizzy or feel intense pain, stop the exercise or adjust your position. I'm a firm believer in working through a degree of pain, since you're getting blood flow to the damaged tissue for healing. Use your best judgment, PLEASE!

4. You can hold each position for as long as you want.

5. In Level 1 Boga, you always have your hands or feet touching the floor. In Level 2 Boga, you're on top of the ball and not touching the floor at all. Level 2 should be done with a spotter or on a pad with some cushion. Again, make sure you've moved all the furniture out of the way.

6. There are resting positions throughout the Boga program. Rest as long as needed, but the faster you get into the next position the more challenging the workout will be.

7. Some of these positions are very challenging. You don't have to attempt every one of them; you can always go back to The Awakening positions.

8. Challenge each other as a family. Kids, see if you can hold the positions longer than Mom and Dad. Mom and Dad, challenge the kids to hold the positions and see if they can beat their best times. Record them in your fitness notebook and reward them if they meet their goals and challenges (such as a bike ride, a hike at the park, or other fun activity that you can do together).

Jim's Boga Fitness Program - The Awakening

Starting Position

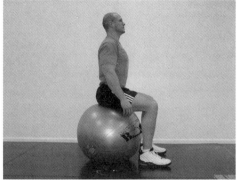

Start by sitting on your ball with perfect posture: abdominals tight, shoulder blades back, arms down to your sides, look straight forward, legs a little wider than shoulder width apart. Extend your arms up, reach up as high as possible stretch all the way through your finger tips and slowly take it down to Rag Doll.

Rag Doll

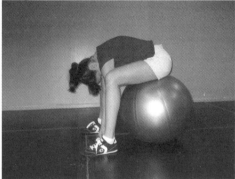

Keep your thighs firm. From your low back to the top of your head, relax and hang out. Let the weight of your head stretch that upper back where all the tension is. Remember, keep your breathing constant. On each exhale, relax and let the spine elongate. This will stretch the muscles from your lower back all the way up to the base of your skull. You may also feel it in the back of your legs.
From Rag Doll, let's go right into Rainbow.

Rainbow

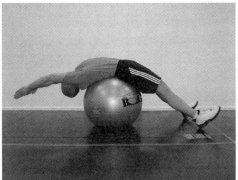

Slowly walk your legs out and lie back on the ball, keeping your legs about 12 to 18 inches apart for a stable base. Straighten your legs out, get on your heels and flex your feet towards you. Reach your arms back and stretch through your finger tips.

Right and Left Side Stretch

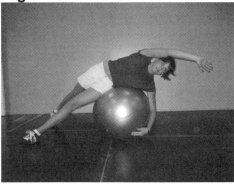

From the Rainbow, roll over to your right hip, keep your legs wide through this transition to prevent rolling off the ball, bring your right leg forward (whatever side you're on, that leg is in front). The more your hip is on top of the ball the better stretch you're going to get. Now, take your left arm over your left ear and reach through your finger tips. Feel the stretch on your side and in your low back. Visualize the blood flow nourishing the discs in your spine. Know that your back is getting stronger. Do the same thing on your left side with your left leg leading.

Tri-Pod

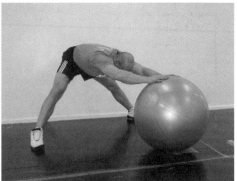

From left side stretch, roll over to your stomach. With the weight of your body on the ball, spread your legs as wide as you can get them. Then roll back onto your forearms to your feet and put your palms on top of the ball, arms straight, and drop your chest down towards the floor. (Make sure your weight is not on the ball. If you move the ball out of the way, you should be able to stay in tri-pod.) Feel the stretch in your inner thighs, low back, chest and shoulders. A fun, full body stretch.

Taurus

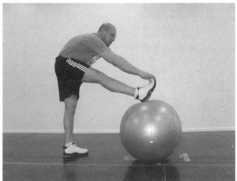

Put your hands as wide as you can get them on the ball and lower down until your stomach rests on the ball. Bring your legs together and push yourself back up and put your right heel on the ball and grab your foot. (If you're not able to grab your foot, reach down as far as you're able). This takes a lot of balance, so be careful. This will stretch out the back of your leg and it's great for the stabilizer muscles for the leg that's on the floor. Switch legs and enjoy the stretch and the progress you're making.

Atlas

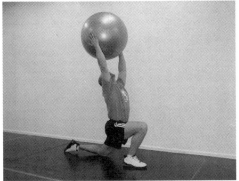

Put your hands as wide as you can get them on the ball and lower yourself down until your stomach rests on the ball. Get down on your knees, grab the ball and take your right foot and step forward. Drop your hips into the floor and take the ball up and back, feel the stretch in the front of your left thigh and in your right gluteus. You also may feel the stretch in your abdominals.

Jackknife

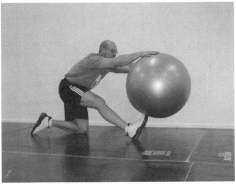

Straighten your right leg out, flex your foot towards you, bend at the hips, put the ball on your toe and feel the stretch in the back of your leg. Try to keep your spine as straight as possible. You can now do your left side. So, you should do the series of right Atlas first, then into right Jackknife, left Atlas then into left Jackknife.

Hammock

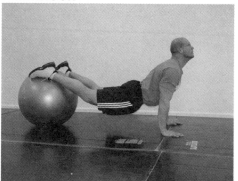

From left Jackknife, put both knees on the floor. Put your body weight on the ball, hands out in front of the ball, and legs shoulder width apart. Now, slowly walk your hands out until your knees are on top of the ball. Squeeze your gluteus maximus (your bottom) and slowly drop your hips towards the floor. Keep your legs straight and firm and keep your arms, chest and shoulders strong. Gently look up and back.

Congratulations, you just learned The Awakening, the warm-up to Jim's Boga Fun Fitness Program. When you complete the Hammock, you can reverse all the positions and eventually get back to the seated positions. Spend anywhere from 10 to 15 minutes doing The Awakening. Memorize the positions and feel free to create your own Awakening. Just make sure you do all positions, so you're sure to stretch out the whole body thoroughly. You can do it everyday as much as you want.

Jim's Boga Fun Fitness Program - Level 1

Let's continue right into the different Boga positions. All positions should flow together; challenge yourself and DIG IN!

Toad

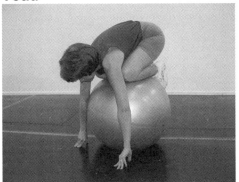

Rest your stomach against the ball, walk out on your hands until your thighs are on the ball, then pull your knees into your chest and sit back on your heels on top of the ball. Once you get used to this position, you will find that it is more of a resting position and a great stretch for your low back as well. If your ball is too big, this position could be difficult.

Table

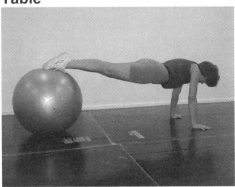

From Toad straighten your legs out then proceed to walk out to the Table. There are many levels of Table. The farther you walk out towards your feet the more difficult it is, so don't try to push yourself too much the first time. Once you get into position, keep your thighs strong, abdominals tight, arms and shoulders firm. Hold, breathe and enjoy! Other options are One Leg Table, or you can Drop a Leaf. Have some fun with this and have someone rest a soft toy or pillow on your back for some fun. You should be able to balance the object if you're holding the position properly. If this bothers your wrists, you can do the position on your forearms. From Table, walk it back to Toad and rest for as long as you needed.

One Leg Table

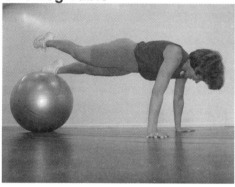

Drop A Leaf Table

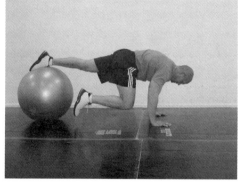

Praying Mantis

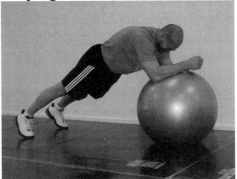

Straighten your legs out, push back and put your feet on the floor and put your forearms on the ball. Make sure your abdominals and thighs are tight, don't let the hips drop down too far and keep your chest off the ball. This is great for your abs. If you aren't challenged, move the ball away from your body.

Oak

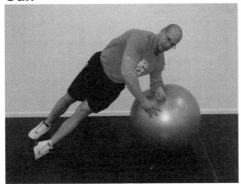

Roll over to your right elbow and put your right leg in front, keep your hips off the ball and legs straight. Little Oak is with your left hand stabilizing the ball, Big Oak is with your left hand off the ball, and Oak Blowing in the Wind is with one leg. All three moves are difficult, but fun! Either roll over on your back or stomach to get into left Oak. In left Oak, keep your left leg forward.

Big Oak

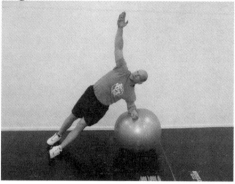

Moon

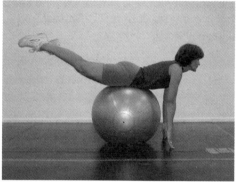

Position yourself so the ball is touching your lower abs to upper thighs, finger tips are all the way back towards the ball, and legs are straight. Now bring your torso and legs up as far as you can. This is one of the best positions for strengthening the low back. Hold, enjoy, then pull it back to Toad and stretch those muscles you just contracted. You can get into Toad after each position if you need a rest or just to stretch.

Z

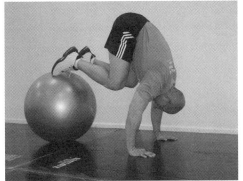

I love the Z. Walk out like you're going to Table. When you get out where your shins are touching the ball, pull your knees into your chest and lift your tail bone up. Just the toes touching is the toughest position. The more your shins touch the ball, the easier the position becomes.

Seal

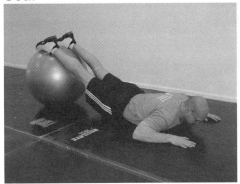

From Z, straighten your legs out to Table and immediately lower yourself down to Seal. Legs are straight, thighs off the ground and enjoy this lower abdominal stretch as you're flexing your lower lumbar.

The Sling Shot - Get Ready

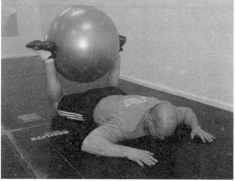

Grab the ball with your legs and curl it back to your gluteus maximus.

The Sling Shot – Aim

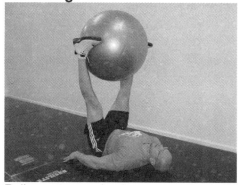

Roll over to your back, squeeze the ball tight and keep your legs straight up.

The Sling Shot – Fire

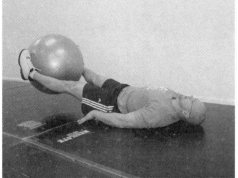

Lower the ball down about 6 to 8 inches from the floor.

Pliers

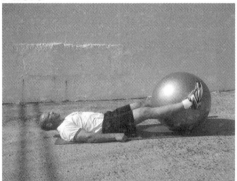

Lie on your back squeezing the ball with your legs. Make sure your legs are directly on each side of the ball and squeeze really tight. This is great for the inner thighs.

Fly

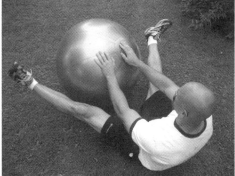

From Pliers, reach your arms up above your chest and slowly sit up until your finger tips are touching the ball and Fly. When you Fly, keep your finger tips on the ball and remove your legs. Keep your legs as straight as possible, bring them up as high as you can and keep your stomach strong. Don't forget to breathe.

The Wedge

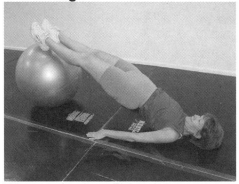

When you're done Flying, bring your legs up and put them on top the ball, slowly lie back down. With a slight bend in your knees and palms on the floor, lift as much of your body off the floor as possible. This is great for your hamstrings, bottom, and low back.

1 Leg Wedge

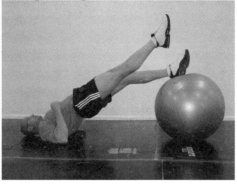

Pikes Peak

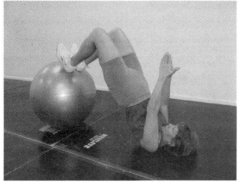

Drop your bottom back down to the floor, bend your knees back to 90 degrees and then make sure your heels are directly on top of the ball. Now lift your hips as high off the floor as possible, making sure your knees are aligned with your hips and shoulders.

Cradle

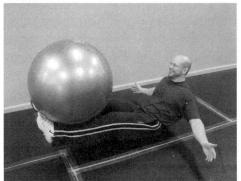

Get back into Pliers. Sit up and put your hands on the ball.
Grab the ball and rest it on your shins.

Shoot The Moon

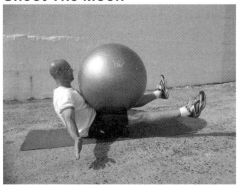

From Cradle, see if you can Shoot the Moon using your legs and
the ball - moving the ball back and forth from your feet to your
chest. Try not to let your heels touch the floor and keep your
back off as well. This one will challenge you.

Check Mark

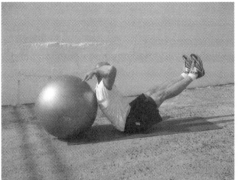

Now grab the ball with your hands, put your feet on the floor and put the ball behind you, so your head and shoulder blades are on the ball. Reach your hands behind your head, put your finger tips on the ball and straighten your legs out and get them as high as you can into the Check Mark. Make sure your shoulder blades aren't touching the ball when you're in Check Mark.

Crab

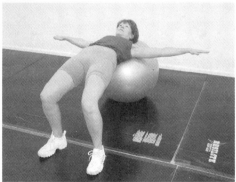

Now you can put your feet on the floor, head and shoulder blades back on the ball and lift your hips up and arms out with your palms up. You're now in Crab! See if you can do One Leg Crab. Don't let those hips drop and keep your head on the ball. See if you can roll it over to Praying Mantis and then push it up to Taurus. This is great for balance and it also is a wonderful stretch for the back of your legs. Don't forget to do both legs!

Rollercoaster

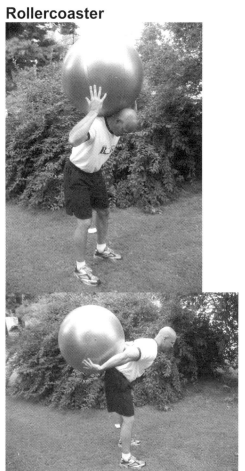

Let's go on a Rollercoaster ride. Grab your ball and lift it over your head and put it on your shoulder blades, bend at the waist, shoulder blades back, then let the ball roll down your back and quickly catch it and bring it underneath you and sit on it. This will likely take some practice. The ball can get away from you, so you may want someone there to catch the ball until you master this one.

Reversal

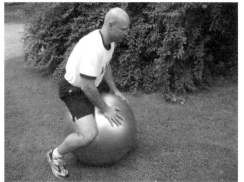

Now that you're sitting on the ball with your shoulder blades back, arms to the side, abdominals as tight as you can get them, take three huge breaths. Get back in the Rag Doll and put your palms on the floor. Straddle the ball and shoot your legs back. That combination is called the Reversal.

Scissors

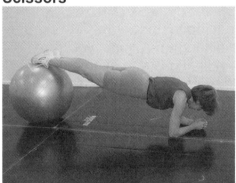

From Reversal, get on your forearms and walk out to the Scissors. This position is great for your abs. Keep your whole body rigid; this is very similar to the Table except you're on your forearms. Feel free to open the Scissors up, lifting one leg off the ball.

Plank

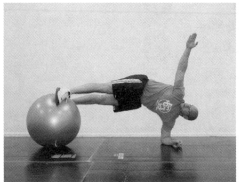

From Scissors, walk it back until your thighs are on the ball. Now you can walk the Plank. Spread your legs out, so you can squeeze the ball with your feet and walk out on your forearms. Bring your left hand up to your finger tips and rotate your torso. This is a hard one, but if you feel daring you can "jump" by bringing that left arm straight up. Don't forget to do both sides. And then get back into Toad.

You don't have to do the positions in this order. After you learn all the different positions, you can make up your own combinations and even create new positions. You should memorize all the positions and once you do you will be able to go through the different combinations without looking at the book. Make up new positions and give them fun names, this can be hours of Fun Fitness for the whole family.

Once you've mastered all the Level 1 Boga positions, you can move on to Level 2. For Level 2, I'm just going to show you the pictures and give you the names of the positions. You can get into Level 2 from the Toad position. Bring your hands up on the ball and move your knees back a little into Cat (see picture). A lot of people who try Cat ask where they should put their knees and hands. That is a hard question to answer. You just have to practice, get on that ball and use every muscle you have to stay on that ball. You're working stabilizer muscles; the more you practice the more those stabilizers will respond. Before you know it, you will master all the Level 2 positions and have great balance. To add variety to the work-out, you can go back and forth from Level 1 to Level 2.

Cat

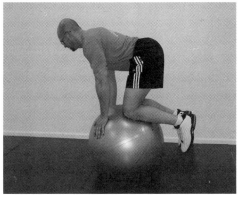

Catcher

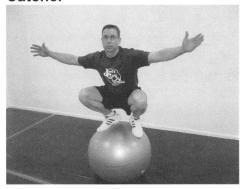

Cliff Hanger

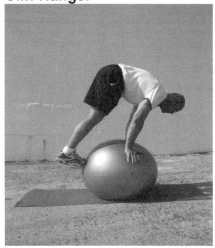

Can Opener

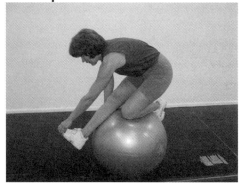

Cannon Ball

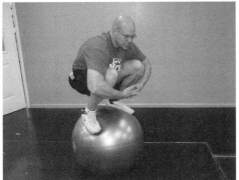

Bear

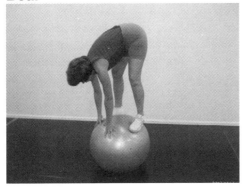

Frog

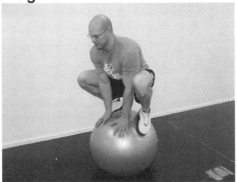

Grasshopper

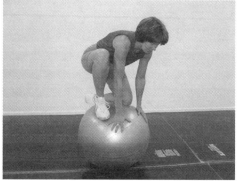

Thinker

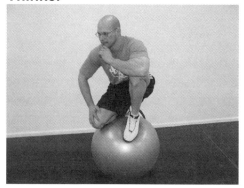

Hurdler

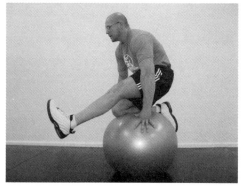

Seat

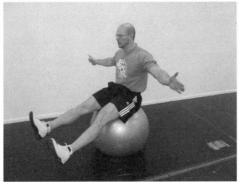

Stand

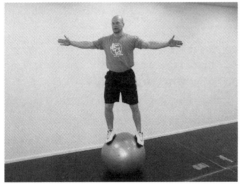

Sky Diver

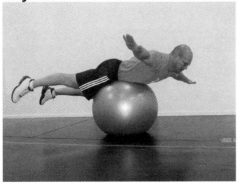

Squat

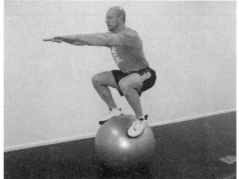

Flamingo

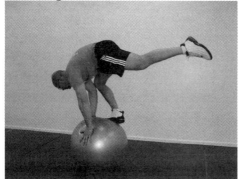

Donkey Kick

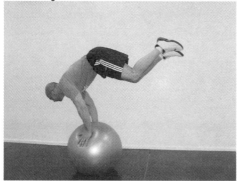

Catapult

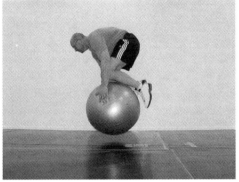

Popcorn

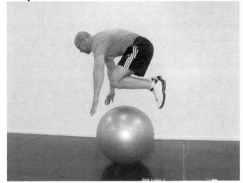

Turtle

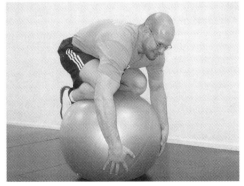

Level 2 Tripod

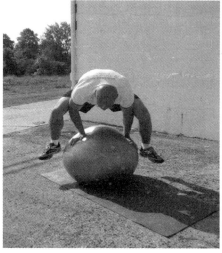

Hare

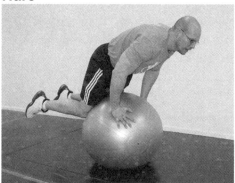

80

Fire Hydrant

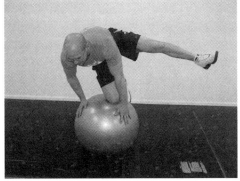

Totem Pole

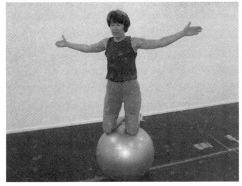

Scorpion

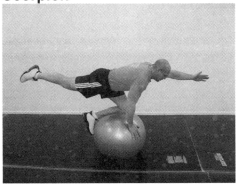

Surfer

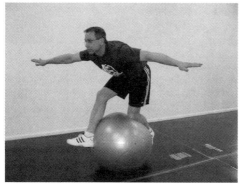

Dragonfly

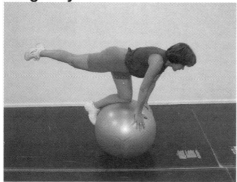

Average Joe

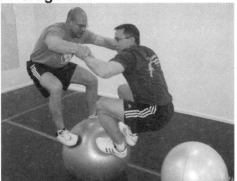

CHAPTER 9

THE FUN FITNESS JUGGLING PROGRAM

I'm hard pressed to find someone out there who wouldn't love to learn to juggle or master a skill toy. I personally love to use skill and juggling toys. I developed a Fun Fitness Program where I incorporate skill juggling toys and physical fitness all in one. There are numerous benefits of learning this skill. Because it's fun, it will motivate and get you excited. And the beauty of it is that you're getting a physical workout and a mental workout as well. I went over the benefits of physical exercise in Chapter 1; now let me briefly go over the benefits of using your brain when you juggle.

Many studies show that juggling can 'boost brain power' and actually make your brain bigger. I don't know about you, but having a little more brain power sounds good to me! *Medical News Today* studied 24 non-jugglers and put them into two groups and assigned one group to practice juggling for three months. The group that didn't juggle showed no difference in brain scans over that period. Those who acquired the skill had an increase in grey matter in two areas of the brain involved in visual and motor activity. Interestingly, this increase in brain size does not last. When the group stopped juggling, they lost the gained brain power and the enhanced regions decreased in size. Dr. Arne May, assistant professor of neurology at the University of Regensburg in Germany says, "the brain is like a muscle, we need to exercise it." *Education World* reports that the juggling program started in Jacksonville schools has helped students concentrate more. For the children who had reading difficulty, it helped improve their reading skills and their overall confidence.

Wow! The Fun Fitness Program you're learning is not only going to make you physically fit, but it may also make you smarter. Not only that, but you'll have quality, fun time you can spend with your family. Are you ready to start? Let's DIG IN!

I'm going to give you basic juggling techniques. You need 3 balls – any balls will do to start, but as you improve you'll want to have balls that are the right weight and size (regulation size juggling balls can be ordered from my website).

Before you start the program, let's go over some basics:

1. First try the 1-ball exercise. Throw the ball from one hand to the other, keeping the ball about forehead level. Make sure the line of travel is an arc, not a circle.

2. The 2-ball exercise. Grab a ball in each hand. Toss the ball in your right hand up to about forehead level and at the top of the arc take the ball in your left hand and toss it to your right hand. Try to do this exercise starting the throw with your left hand also. Practice this exercise until you can do both ways smoothly. Make sure you don't throw both balls at the same time or throw the balls in a circle.

3. 3-ball exercise. If you're right handed, hold 2 balls in your right hand, and 1 in your left. If you're a lefty, put them both in your left hand and one in your right. Start by throwing the ball

in the front of your right hand in an arc about forehead high to your left hand. When the ball reaches its highest point, take the ball in your left hand and throw it in an arc to your right hand. Just like the 2-ball exercise. When the ball thrown from your left hand reaches the arc, throw the ball from your right hand in an arc to your left hand, and so on….

This is a basic lesson on how to juggle. This pattern is one of the most popular which is called the cascade. Don't get frustrated if you keep dropping the balls, because we are now going into our Fun Fitness Program where dropping the balls is going to benefit you (think the big O! Optimism)! I'm excited, so let's have a big smile and continue.

Fun Fitness Juggling

There are four levels to my Fun Fitness Juggling Program. They are all very beneficial, but each higher one challenges you a little more. The concept is very simple. Every time you drop a ball, you get to do a combination of exercises before picking the balls up to continue. It doesn't matter how many balls you drop; you still just owe yourself that one particular combination of exercises. If you're a beginner juggler you might want to use 1 ball and just throw it back and forth. Or do the 2 ball exercise and master that. Remember, this isn't just to learn how to juggle. This is a physical workout as well, so when you drop a ball, welcome that. Get excited, because you now get to do your physical exercises.

Level 1 Fun Fitness Juggling

So let's start with Level 1. When you drop a ball, you owe yourself 2 fun lunges (1 on each leg) and 1 fun squat.

Lunge

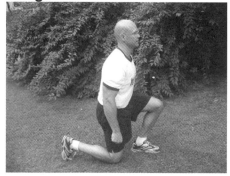

Squat

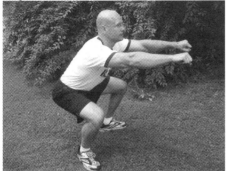

Those two movements work the biggest muscles in the body; therefore, you are burning a lot of calories, getting your heart rate up, and releasing endorphins that give you a sense of well being and joy! Why people use drugs to alter their state I'll never figure out, when you can get this natural healthy high from Fun Fitness Juggling.

I'm not the best juggler; I'm getting a lot better, (I apply my 5 "STEPP" success program to just about anything I do in life and it works!) but I still drop the balls a lot. I've pretty much mastered the cascade, so I can do that a while before I drop a ball. But can I take a ball behind my back with my right hand on a consistent basis without dropping them? No! In a one half hour period, I did nearly 150 lunges and squats, I worked up a great sweat, and my brain got bigger too! (Hey kids, use this one on your parents. When Mom calls you inside, you can say, "In a minute Mom, I'm juggling and increasing the grey matter in my brain - just trying to get smarter Mom!") If you feel like all you're doing is lunging and squatting and not getting any better at juggling, you can go to the squat option only. Just don't bend at the waist to pick up the balls when you drop them. I call that the lackadaisical way to pick up something and you don't want to be lackadaisical! Squat your bottom down low, bend at the hips and knees; it's better for your back and you'll learn to pick things up properly. Don't stay with the single squat too long. As soon as your juggling improves, immediately incorporate the lunges.

You can do Level 1 Fun Fitness Juggling program everyday for at least a half an hour. If at first you can't do it that long, start with 5 or 10 minutes, and add a couple minutes each day. Shoot for a TARGET.   By the end of the month, you could be up to 60 minutes. Aim high! I'll do Level 1 for hours, especially if I have the time on a sunny afternoon at the park with my family.

Level 2 Fun Fitness Juggling

OK, are you ready to pick it up a notch, DIG IN a little more? Good, let's do it. The only thing different from Level 1 to Level 2 is when you drop the ball (or balls) you reward yourself with 5 pushups, 20 runners, 2 fun lunges and 1 fun squat. Let's talk about the good old-fashioned push-up, one of the best exercises ever for full body strength. Not too many people do the form properly. Hands should be a little wider than shoulder width apart and feet about the same. Your hands should be parallel with your chest. At first, put one of the balls right below your chest so you gently touch it every time down. One more thing, your body should be rigid. Don't let those hips sag; you should almost have a straight line from shoulder to hip to knee to ankle. Now that's a push up!   If regular ones are too challenging, drop to your knees and use the same principles.

Push-Up

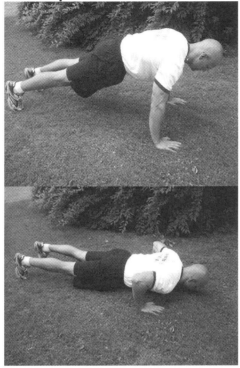

Right from that 5th push-up, go into 20 runners.

Runner

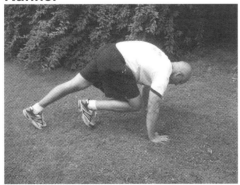

Alternate your legs and bring your knees into your chest, 10 each way. Advanced runners are when you bring your knees into your chest without letting your foot touch the floor. Stand up immediately and do your 2 fun lunges and 1 fun squat. This gets challenging, especially if you're dropping the balls often. Create your own workout. You can go back and forth between Level 1 and 2. Alternate levels every time you drop a ball. Or do Level 1 for a half hour then finish off fifteen minutes with Level two. No matter what you do, do the Fun Fitness Juggling Program with ENTHUSIASM. And please, don't get frustrated if you drop balls constantly. With PATIENCE and PERSEVERANCE, you will eventually become a great juggler as you're getting in great shape.

Level 3 Fun Fitness Juggling

Are you ready to tackle Level 3? Good! Let's make it happen. This time when you drop a ball you owe yourself: 5 squat jump-outs, 5 to 10 push-ups, 10 alternate standing kicks, 2 fun lunges and 1 fun squat. You can really get your heart pumping doing Level 3.

Squat Jump-Outs

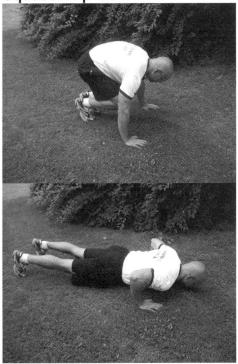

When you do the jump-outs, squat all the way down placing your palms on the floor. Your knees should be between your arms. Then, jump both feet out. Keep your abdominals as tight as possible when your feet hit. Immediately jump your feet back to you, tucking the knees into the chest and stand up. When you stand up, throw your chest out and squeeze your shoulder blades together and immediately repeat the exercise. You literally contract nearly every muscle in the body when you do this movement.

Alternate Standing Kicks

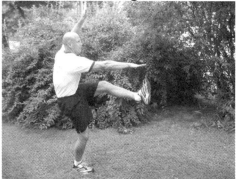

Now let me explain the alternate standing kicks. Stand with your arms above your head. Kick your right foot up as high as you can as you bring your left arm down and see if you can touch your toe. Repeat on the other side. Make sure you keep your leg as straight as possible and bring your arms back up high and strong every time. Now you can finish with your two fun lunges and one fun squat.

This is a great, fun work-out to do with your children. Parents, you have to take the initiative and practice this work-out yourself. You can do this program anywhere. Then, you can have hours of fun with your children teaching and learning a skill together as you're getting physically fit. Get enthusiastic about it; enthusiasm and excitement are contagious. If you're excited, your children will want to participate. They will feel they are missing out if they don't do the Fun Fitness Juggling Program.

Any Skill Toy Will Do
You can do The Fun Fitness Juggling Program with any skill toy. I use juggling sticks and diabolos (can be purchased at www.funfitnesscoach.com).

This adds variety to your exercise program. Stay with the same format: every time you drop a stick or diabolo, either do level 1, 2, or 3. Before you know it, you and your children will be having hours of Fun Fitness.

Level 4 Fun Fitness Juggling - Fun Fitness Juggling Boga Program

My last Fun Fitness Juggling Program is advanced and takes a lot of balance and hand/eye coordination. Like all the other programs, it is loads of fun. To begin, you'll need to master the Totem Pole, which is a Level 2 Jim's Boga move with just your knees on the ball. The Totem Pole is great for your thighs and builds core strength and balance.

Start by holding one juggling ball and get into Totem Pole. Then, throw the juggling ball back and forth; remember to throw it in an arc at about forehead level. Once you start tossing the ball, you'll notice you really have to concentrate to stay balanced on the exercise ball. If you happen to drop the juggling ball or fall off the exercise ball, you owe yourself a Praying Mantis Roll-Out.

Get into the Praying Mantis, with your forearms on the ball and your abs tight. Then roll the ball out as far as you can without letting your hips drop. Do a set of 10. This can be challenging. If you can't roll the ball out without feeling some unnatural pressure in your low back, just hold the Praying Mantis for 5 to 10 inhales. When you're done, grab your juggling ball and roll into Toad, then Cat, and then into Totem Pole again. On the second drop or fall, get right into Oak and do an Oak Roll-Out. You'll find you don't have to roll the ball out very far before it gets challenging. You can do this in Big Oak, Little Oak, or Oak Blowing in the Wind. Keep your hips and abs rigid. Don't let those hips drop at all when you roll that ball out. Remember to do both sides, 10 each way. Get back into Totem Pole and on the third drop get into the Z and do a set of 10 Z Roll-Outs. The Z Roll-Out is going from Z to Table. These are the three Boga moves I use in Level 4; keep repeating these three moves. When you master the Totem Pole and one ball, add 2 or 3 juggling balls and continue the program. Now you're juggling as you're kneeling on a ball. Keep practicing and don't give up. You can do anything!

Five Effective ½ Hour Workouts
(These can be done every day or at least three times a week)
Workout 1:

       15 minutes Level 1 Fun Fitness Juggling
       15 minutes Level 2 Fun Fitness Juggling

Workout 2:

       10 minutes Level 1 Fun Fitness Juggling
       10 minutes Level 2 Fun Fitness Juggling
       10 minutes Level 3 Fun Fitness Juggling

Workout 3:

       10 minutes Level 1 Fun Fitness Juggling
       20 minutes Jim's Boga

Workout 4:

       20 minutes Jim's Boga (first 5 minutes do The Awakening)
       5 minutes Level 2 Fun Fitness Juggling
       5 minutes Level 3 Fun Fitness Juggling

Workout 5:

      30 minutes Level 1, 2, and 3 Fun Fitness
      Juggling (rotate levels every time you
      drop a ball)

Five Effective 1 Hour Workouts
(These can be done every day or at least three times
a week)

Workout 1:

      20 minutes Level 1 Fun Fitness Juggling
      20 minutes Level 2 Fun Fitness Juggling
      20 minutes Level 1 Fun Fitness Juggling

Workout 2:

      30 minutes Jim's Boga (first 10 minutes
      do The Awakening)
      10 minutes Level 1 Fun Fitness Juggling
      10 minutes Level 2 Fun Fitness Juggling
      10 minutes Level 3 Fun Fitness Juggling

Workout 3:

      10 minutes Level 1 Fun Fitness Juggling
      10 minutes Jim's Boga
      10 minutes Level 2 Fun Fitness Juggling
      10 minutes Jim's Boga
      10 minutes Level 3 Fun Fitness Juggling
      10 minutes Jim's Boga

Workout 4:

      20 minutes Level 1 Fun Fitness Juggling
      20 minutes Level 2 Fun Fitness Juggling
      20 minutes Level 3 Fun Fitness Juggling

Workout 5:

      30 minutes Jim's Boga (first 10 minutes
      do The Awakening)
      15 minutes Level 2 Fun Fitness Juggling
      15 minutes Level 3 Fun Fitness Juggling

Feel free to extend the workout longer than the duration prescribed. You can also create your own combinations. Challenge yourself and have a great time at your Fun Fitness Program. Please don't get frustrated if you keep dropping your juggling balls; welcome the drop, because you get to do the physical portion of the workout. If you're juggling or doing your push-ups, you're getting major benefits either way, so have fun!

Other Work-Out Ideas
I encourage you to find other activities that you can do as a family to continue the fun. Some additional ideas are listed below:

1. Walk, walk, walk. Spend quality time talking to your children while you're walking. Go to the mall, go through the neighborhood, go to nature trails, etc. Create a family ritual of going for evening walks. Get the younger kids out of the stroller and have them walk. Don't put them in the shopping cart at stores either; let them walk.

2. Ride bikes together. Children love to ride bicycles – need I say more?

3. Play (active) games with your children. Don't remember the rules to Ghosts in the Graveyard? Check out www.gameskidsplay.net for information and ideas.

4. Go to the park. Parents, don't just sit on a bench to watch; play with them.

5. Set up an obstacle course in the backyard. Get creative and have fun. Use a stopwatch and see if kids can beat their best time. You'll be amazed at the number of neighborhood kids and adults who want to give the course a try.

6. Have a dance party. Introduce your children to the dance tunes popular in your high school days.

7. Do yard work together. Planting and pulling weeds, raking leaves, shoveling snow, etc. Incorporate a game into the task and have fun - make piles of leaves in which to jump, have a snow ball fight, etc.

8. Join an exercise class. Have you always wanted to learn how to tap dance? Show your children that learning and exercising are fun at all ages.

9. Send your children on a treasure hunt. Have each clue give directions for moving to the next clue, such as hopping, skipping, or running to the next location.

10. Do seasonal activities: run through puddles, go swimming, jump in leaf piles, go sledding or ice skating.

CHAPTER 10

Make The Change Today

I hope this book has inspired and motivated you to embark on an exercise program and healthy, moderate eating lifestyle. Make the change today; don't wait. Help encourage your family members to join your Fun Fitness Program. Reread the "5 STEPP" success program over and over again and memorize the Fun Fitness Program. Bodies were meant to move, so make the commitment and nourish your body with balanced nutrition. You will be "Fit to Achieve" all of your biggest dreams. I'm rooting for you! I want you to succeed and I know you will.

Call or e-mail and let me know how your program is going. Please share your success stories with me and your experience may be incorporated into another book. I'd love to hear from you!

Sincerely,
Jim
America's Fun Fitness Coach
419-420-7586
www.funfitnesscoach.com
funfitnesscoach@woh.rr.com